Dropping Weight Just With Walking

How Walking Changed My Life

Ann Vase

kind are declared or implied. Readers acknowledge that the author is not engaged in the rendering of legal, financial, medical or professional advice. The content within this book has been derived from various sources. Please consult a licensed professional before attempting any techniques outlined in this book.

By reading this document, the reader agrees that under no circumstances is the author responsible for any losses, direct or indirect, that are incurred as a result of the use of the information contained within this document, including, but not limited to, errors, omissions, or inaccuracies.

Table of Contents

Introduction

  Goal Setting

    Motion Produces Self-Esteem

Chapter 1: Running vs. Walking

  Run or Walk for Weight Loss?

  Walk for Burning Fat

Chapter 2: Get Ready and Stay Ready

  Avoid Making Excuses

    Should I Consult With My Doctor?

Chapter 3: Get Those Muscles Working

  Stretching

  Arm Training While Walking

Chapter 4: Walking Plan

  Changing Walking Speed

  What About Walking on a Treadmill?

Chapter 5: Shedding Pounds

  Implementing the Diet

  What About Eating out?

Chapter 6: The Power of Water in Weight Loss

Tips to up Your Daily Water Intake

Do I Need to Drink Just Water?

Walking Has Changed My Life

Dropping Weight Just With Walking

How Walking Changed My Life

Introduction

Are you fed up with how you feel every single day? Exhausted, overstressed, in constant pain, drained of energy. Does all that sound familiar? Then it is time to make a change. A sedentary lifestyle takes its toll on you, whether you realize it or not, so give a pledge to stop this vicious cycle and start moving. It doesn't have to be elaborate or demand tons of skills and resources, on the contrary, go for something that is easy as pie and so liberating that it won't even feel like working out.

Walking is a fundamental instinct for humans. You will be amazed at the awesome benefits it can offer you long-term. The best part? It doesn't require anything other than a clear road ahead and your will to change. Step by step, you feel your muscles burn and you start shaping your dream body and before you know it, the dream becomes reality (Harvard Health Publishing, 2018). Of course, Rome wasn't built in a day, so you cannot expect your body to adjust overnight and start craving for more exercise. But it will happen, trust me. Sooner than later, you will be counting backwards till your next walking session.

"There are many other forms of exercise, so why choose walking?" This is one of the many questions people ask me. Honestly, for me there is no comparison. Walking is the only workout that you can do no matter who you are, no matter where you are or what you are wearing. It doesn't matter if you have some extra pounds (or more than a few dozens), if you have been working out your whole life or if you have never taken up sports before. All you have to do is move your feet. But before you thrive through striding, it is time to set your own personalized goals.

Goal Setting

Let's face it, things will not always go as planned and the journey will not always be easy. In fact, you should expect bumps along the way, so does that mean that it is not worth it? On the contrary! It is definitely one of the most important decisions that you will make in your entire life. But you need some motivation that keeps you going, and this is where you need to focus before anything else. Goal setting is the first step prior to successfully adopting a new behavioral pattern. Envision how you want your life to turn out and then devote your life into making this vision a reality. Does that make sense?

Goal setting is a process that takes time and effort. Consider what it is that you wish to achieve. Define every step of the way, so that nothing can intimidate you in the process. Read all about what you are supposed to do while working out, how you can optimize your performance and enjoy the best experience. After that, think of all the obstacles and how to overcome them. Above all, be sure to envision all the benefits that will come from this shift in your life. What good will that do to your health, your mood, your future? These are all great things to keep in mind, preventing you from jumping the rails and steering away from your target.

In order to commit to your plan, it is best to write everything down. This will hold you accountable, although you do get a second chance, and a third and a fourth one along the way. If you think you can work out at a specific pace and be comfortable with that, then this is your first goal. Be sure to report back and evaluate your plan. You might have overestimated your power or maybe it is time to push further. There is nothing static about it, only progress and bliss. If there's something that does not click, then let it go. Modify your sessions, according to what you like and what you don't. You will certainly come up with great ideas if you think outside the box. Don't hold back and stay positive!

Motion Produces Self-Esteem

Positivity means everything, especially when you are about to embark on a challenging journey to wellness. If you feel overwhelmed by negative emotions and always fear for the worst, then you are bound to experience just that. This is a phenomenon called the "self-fulfilling prophecy," which confirms what you have been expecting to happen in life. So, guess what? If you think negatively, then chances are that this is what you are going to get. Don't prepare yourself for failure. This kind of mentality will only lead you to disappointment, so it is counter-productive. By being positive about the outcome of your endeavors, you expect that good things will happen in the end. This allows you some peace of mind and motivates you to try even harder.

You don't need to beat yourself up, when something goes wrong. You are only human and humans have the tendency to stray from the plan, acting on impulses and regretting things they have done. However, this is not a sprint. It is a marathon and you are in it for the long run, so it matters to persist in what you do and go on until you are there. And through this process, you will only feel more empowered and filled with self-esteem. It is your accomplishment, after all.

The more you move, the more you will become hooked to the process of moving. You will no longer anticipate the time when you sit around and relax. Instead, you will be looking forward to going out and walking. This is your chance to focus on your inner self, elaborate on what has happened throughout the day. During your workout, you can listen to your favorite songs or even a self-improvement session. You can fill your lungs with fresh air or catch up with a good friend, as you both enjoy your brisk stroll, because movement is what brings people together, in the end.

Chapter 1: Running vs. Walking

It doesn't take a rocket scientist to understand the amazing benefits that derive from exercise. You were meant to move around rather than stay still. "A rolling stone gathers no moss" according to an old proverb. Since motion is in your DNA, you should have no problem incorporating it into your daily routine. Start slow and gradually push yourself. You will notice a significant difference in the way you feel and look early on—even from the first couple of days.

Running and walking are both excellent forms of cardiovascular workout options. They help you shed those extra pounds and keep them off, by burning calories and boosting your metabolism at a much faster rate than if you just sat still. Furthermore, they both assist you in shaping up by increasing your stamina and getting fit. Aesthetics aside, running and walking contribute a great deal to the improvement of your health state, empowering your heart. If this is not enough, other benefits include better quality of sleep and enhanced overall immune system. Now that we have clarified just how vital it is to incorporate cardio into your daily lifestyle, what should you actually choose?

It goes without even saying that running burns twice as many calories as walking. Surely it takes more effort to run and therefore the difference is perfectly justifiable. On the other hand, walking is much easier to implement. Well, sometimes the key to success lies in simplicity, and what is simpler than walking? Your first true milestone in life will certainly improve your overall health and wellness, and you can increase the calories that you burn, through elevating the speed of walking or even through adding extra weight or choosing an inclined path rather than a smooth, even road.

Another thing that you need to remember is that running comes with a greater risk of getting injured. This makes sense, since running means that you put more pressure on your joints and muscles to keep up with the challenges, so if you are a newbie, then you should think twice prior to pushing yourself to the limits by running. This could lead to hairline fractures (also known as stress fractures), knee and back pain, joint pain and of course, sprained ankles and shin splints. These health risks seem to be increasing, if you are carrying a lot of weight and/or if you are totally new in this kind of lifestyle. Professional athletes or people who have been running their whole life will react much differently than the way inexperienced people without any serious physical activity background will.

There are fans of both workouts, for sure. People who have been exercising for long prefer running, since they have already become used to such a routine. In addition, they feel like they are getting more bang for the buck. This means that they firmly believe that through running, their efforts pay out more than in any other form of exercise. Unlike running, walking can serve as recreational and therefore it is frowned upon by some. It is not rare for people to doubt that walking can be defined as a workout to begin with.

Nonetheless, the versatility of walking is second to none. Even an older person recovering from surgery can take up walking and improve their life significantly. Starting at a young age and covering all age groups, it feels that anyone can join in. Walking does not put so much strain to the body, which is great, especially for beginners in the thrilling world of exercise. It is needless to say that a newbie's chances of doing more harm than good during running are much higher than they are while walking.

So, in a nutshell, nobody will argue with the acknowledgement that both running and walking can work wonders for you. However, you need to be realistic and select the type of exercise that makes the most out of your effort, without putting your body and health at risk. In case you have never been committed to working out regularly, walking is the best option to start shaping up. It offers all the outstanding benefits, without the annoying downsides that might spoil all the fun for you.

Run or Walk for Weight Loss?

When weight loss is on the table, things may change a little bit. Running or walking? This dilemma is real. As mentioned earlier, running leads to more calories being burned. Still, is this the only variable to take into consideration? Certainly not. And although nobody claims that running is bad for you, in the end you will see that walking has its own unique selling points, making it an amazing competitor.

First of all, walking is for everybody. You can stride without first having exercised a minute in your life. And this is great, particularly since many people lacking confidence do not choose to join the local gym. That way, they wouldn't have to be in a situation that may potentially embarrass them. Through walking, however, they can build their stamina and muscles, while at the same time building their confidence and self-esteem.

Walking is a wonderful way to get out of the house and be outdoors, which is vital for dieters. If you torture yourself constantly thinking of food and if you are on the verge of giving up and giving in, just go out for a walk. As a result, you will benefit yourself both ways. You will burn more calories and you will get distracted, possibly preventing an episode of overeating. Of course, you can go out for a run— but walking just feels more doable, especially when such a decision is made in the spur of the moment. Besides, you can engage in walking for longer than running, so the more the time spent outdoors, the more the chances you won't fall off the wagon with your diet.

From everything that has been pointed out above, there is no mystery. Both running and walking provide exceptional benefits when it comes to losing weight. But if you are a novice in working out and you want to enjoy a sustainable, easy and versatile form of exercise, then walking should be your number one option. It will give you the energy you need, as well as help you burn the fat off and distract you when you feel like you'll fall into bad habits again.

Walk for Burning Fat

Burning fat is the goal of working out, right? So wouldn't it be a pity to find out that your walking routine doesn't pay out as anticipated? This is why you need to know how to maximize the fat-burning benefits of walking. As a consequence, you will be able to burn more calories and increase your metabolism rate significantly. And of course, this all leads to burning fat and shedding those extra pounds.

Firstly, you must prolong your walking workout for as long as possible. The more you walk, the better the results. But since this is not an option for many people (since time is money), there are more tips you can use. For instance, you can try working faster and pushing yourself to follow a harder path than usual. Then, you can add small breaks into your routine to mix it up a little.

Using the stairs can be a wonderful way to maximize your fat burning machine. When you walk, spot the stairs nearby and try to squeeze them in your walking session. The same goes for hills that make you put more effort to walk. It doesn't have to be a lengthier walking route, as long as it is a more challenging one.

Finally, this is something that you might not have considered until now. You can use walking poles, even if you think that they are only suitable for walking in the mountains or so. The truth is that these poles will allow you to walk faster and more intensely, without even realizing it. Walking with the aid of walking poles is otherwise known as Nordic walking, with a direct reference to the spectacular landscapes of the North in Europe. Basically, what you do is to make your arm swings a lot more intense, due to the use of the poles. Simple enough, yet so fun!

Chapter 2: Get Ready and Stay Ready

"Well begun is half done" and therefore you ought to be thoroughly prepared before setting out on your walking challenge. Determination will boost your self-confidence and provide you with everything you require for a successful future in walking. Plus, having planned ahead will give you the "thumbs-up" to overcome any obstacle that gets in the way. Otherwise, you will most likely waste time trying to figure out how to cope with an unexpected situation.

You don't need fancy equipment or expensive subscriptions to successfully indulge in walking. What you need is the right mood, along with comfortable clothes and shoes. You should avoid jeans at all costs! Instead, choose lightweight pants that are able to absorb the sweat and keep you dry during your workout. A sweater or T-shirt (depending on the weather) is just fine, although typically you can wear whatever makes you feel good and comfortable. Avoid fabrics that are too tight and do not let your body breathe. Above anything else, make sure that your clothes actually fit you. The same goes for the shoes that you select to wear, since they will improve your walking performance a great deal. There are also specialized items that you can choose to buy at quite affordable prices. For instance, you can use protective wraps for your feet or even ankle braces. Particularly if you have been injured and now you are recovering, these products will make a huge difference and enable you to get back on track.

Of course, a motivating playlist and maybe some good company will complete the missing pieces and offer you the perfect walking experience. You can listen to some music or even a podcast on your phone to entertain you! Then, you can enrich your equipment with the purchase of a solid fitness tracker. Wearables can be extremely helpful to those, who wish to track their progress and check their heart rate, how many calories they have burned and the speed at which they walk. A pedometer or step tracker, a smartwatch or an app on your phone will do the trick.

A bottle of water or energy drink to replenish electrolytes, a dry towel, an extra outfit you can wear after your exercise is over, a light treat you can snack on, a hat and sunglasses or a waterproof jacket, all these elements should be under your consideration. But the final combo is up to you. Are you intrigued? Then stay tuned and find out how you can use walking to lose weight easy and fast, staying healthy and fit. Get those sneakers on and let's do it!

Avoid Making Excuses

Getting ready for walking doesn't always mean that you don't need to figure out things to do. On the contrary, finding out more about things to avoid makes a lot of sense. Moreover, you should be aware of what might come along the way and prevent you from reaching your walking goals. In this way, you will indeed be ready and deal with these negative situations from the start, and what could be more negative than a good old excuse, which is meant to get you out of establishing your new routine?

Let's face it, there are many excuses you can use. Since the beginning of time, these are the most commonly used excuses for you to avoid like the plague:

- "I am exhausted, my feet are killing me, I don't have the energy to walk"
- "After working all day, the only thing I want to do is rest, not walk"
- "I am too old, so walking is not viable for me on a regular basis"
- "I feel lonely when walking"
- "It is so boring to walk as a form of exercise, nothing special about that"
- "It is too hot outside for walking"

- "Well, it is too cold outside for walking"
- "Hm, it's raining outside, so I won't go walking"

What do you feel about these excuses? Do they make sense? Would you imagine yourself using them in a way that keeps you away from your goals? I imagine that it can be tempting to indulge in such excuses, and a lot of these statements are actually valid, since you will most likely be tired and indeed, weather conditions may affect your walking experience.

Nevertheless, you need to train your mind in overcoming the obstacles that come your way, because these excuses come from obstacles that have appeared before you and you want to cope with them. But it is essential that you develop defensive mechanisms that allow you to endure and stick with your plan to walk. The weather is not going to be perfect every day. There will be sunshine, as much as sudden rainfall or too much cold or even extreme heat that threatens to compromise your walking session. Will you let that happen?

By preparing for all occasions, you automatically eliminate the possibility of getting caught off guard. As a result, you will keep up with your plan and nothing will stop you. For instance, if you don't have time to walk because you are babysitting, why don't you take the children with you? You can enjoy some quality time together and still get your cardio for the day. On the other hand, if it is too hot outside, then be sure to stay hydrated and don't wear too much, preferably light clothing and always wear sunscreen. In fact, a great alternative would be to find somewhere to walk indoors. A gym, a track field, or even a shopping mall can do the trick for you.

I cannot stress enough how important it is to have the right shoes for you. Walking with the wrong shoes can be disastrous, meaning that you may injure yourself and perform worse than anticipated. If you are experiencing any pain or discomfort, or if you feel like you are too old to walk as a form of exercise, then you should consult with your doctor. And get ready to add some spice into the mix to avoid getting bored or lonely. There are solutions, if you have the right attitude.

Should I Consult With My Doctor?

Another growing concern related to taking up a hobby that features physical activity is that of health issues emerging along the way. Generally, it is good to check your health status before changing your lifestyle by incorporating regular exercise. On the bright side, walking is pretty much the safest workout you can choose, even if you suffer from health problems. It is no wonder why doctors all over the world instruct their patients to start walking at a brisk pace twice to three times per week, at least. However, if you have an underlying health condition like diabetes type 1 and 2, heart disease, or even high blood pressure, it is a must that you consult with your doctor first.

Even if you don't visit your doctor prior to starting out your workout routine, it is imperative that you do if you notice any symptoms that alarm you. If you feel dizzy or lightheaded, if you experience pain or swelling, if you notice that your heart beats too fast, then go to the doctor. He will suggest tweaking your workout sessions a bit or going on as planned, depending on the diagnosis. Obviously, medical tests aim mainly at determining whether or not your body is strong enough to encounter the challenges of working out, especially with regards to your heart.

One thing to point out, though, is that you should not overestimate your powers and think that you are invincible. For example, if you have started to experience moderate pain in the joints or a bit of swelling in the ankles, then there is no room for speculation. Seek medical assistance so that you are well aware of what is happening. And in any case, even the slightest doubt on your behalf should lead to a visit to your doctor. Better safe than sorry, wouldn't you say   so?

Chapter 3: Get Those Muscles Working

The first step is always the hardest. All this planning, studying and anticipating can be exhausting. But there comes a time when you have to take a stand and move forward. There is no room for delays. Don't postpone the beginning of your journey to walking bliss. As you will come to realize, this might be the biggest decision of your life. Through a simple form of exercise like walking, new horizons appear in the distance. Even if you start slow, it doesn't really matter. As long as you are consistent in your efforts, your life will change, so get those muscles working for improving your wellness beyond your wildest dreams.

By the way, do you actually know which muscles will be working, every step you take? Obviously, you cannot expect to tone up your entire body, there are solutions that allow you to do so, as you will get to see later on. But for now, you concentrate on your lower body. Glutes, quadriceps and hamstrings, tibialis anterior and posterior, soleus, gastrocnemius and the peroneals, along with hip flexors all work together. Some of them sound funny, I give you that. Nevertheless, they join forces, in order to assist you in your walking sessions.

So how can you tone up your muscles and strengthen them? How can you energize them, make them more flexible and enable them to perform way better than before? One answer to this question is through stretching! As you will get to see, stretching has been gravely misunderstood. It has multiple benefits and it can be used for various purposes. Aren't you excited?

Stretching

Why is stretching so important? Well, think about it this way. Your muscles tend to shrink and tighten over time. Unless you give them the care they are entitled to, they become less and less flexible. This leads to achy attempts to move around and activate them. Of course, since they are just coming out of their hibernation, it makes total sense why they are reacting like that. However, if you wake them up gently and if you persist in keeping them involved, they will reward you with flexibility beyond your wildest dreams!

This is what stretching is all about. Making your muscles stronger, longer and more flexible so as to help you out with your day challenges. The main types of stretching are static and dynamic ones. The former is probably the most popular type, with extensions of your body parts to target specific muscles. This is where you reach to grab your toes and feel the muscles burning. The lunge is a perfect example of dynamic stretching. Of course, both these types are beneficial to your body—provided that you know how and when to engage in either one of them.

Unfortunately, there are many misconceptions as far as stretching is concerned. Even professionals will advise you not to start working out before having completed at least the basic stretching exercises. But is this true? They claim that it is like diving in the crystal cold waters, without having first dipped your feet in to adjust to the temperature. Have you ever felt that? The shock that runs through your body?

Well, that could not be further from the truth, I am afraid! In fact, your body is still cold. By engaging in stretching, you simply tire your muscles and tendons during your workout. As a result, your athletic performance declines and you do not even prevent injuries—as I said, your body is cold, so no impact there. If you want to benefit your body prior to workouts, then you have to warm up by starting slow. As a consequence, your body will get ready for the "main course" and ease itself into more intense exercise.

Stretching after a workout is a whole different situation. Its main benefit is muscle recovery. Through these amazingly simple yet effective exercises, your blood flows smoothly, thus muscle damage is decreased and better managed. Plus, your nervous system must relax and stretching is the best way to do that. And if you still need some convincing, how about the impact of stretching on your heart health? Stretching allows your heart to slow down and take it easy, so no more stress!

Arm Training While Walking

Walking offers amazing results, but it is true that this form of exercise mainly focuses on the lower body. On the bright side, you can twist your routine a little bit and get a complete workout. Without using any weights, you can add some repetitive moves using your arms for the perfect combo. The reason for not using any weights is that they will be slowing you down while they do not actually help you burn more calories or tone up as much. Anyway, these moves will help you tone up your chest and arms, improving your posture and shaping up your tummy and back. They are easy to incorporate, simple and they do not require any special equipment.

Let's see how you can engage in arm training while walking. These sets of exercises target the upper body, which is a bit left out in comparison with the lower body during walking sessions. First off, you can swing your arms while bending them, keeping your tummy engaged. Move the arms back and forth in turn, as if you were trying to push your body forward. A bust lift is an excellent form of exercise that you can add to your walking routine, so as to tone your upper body. You simply lift your arms with the elbows reaching the height of your shoulders. Bring them together, so the two elbows can touch each other in front of your chin and then repeat.

Getting your arms up and down over your head while walking is another great option. Just make sure that you complete sets of these repetitive moves, to get the optimal results. Even if you don't move, however, you can cross your arms in front of your chest and walk like that. It allows you to strengthen your waist and back, while at the same time pushing you forward and increasing your walking speed. Last but not least, you can play with your arms and get great benefits, while entertaining yourself. For instance, if you lift your arms in front of your chest and make fists, then you can pretend that you are throwing punches like you would in boxing. In this way, it does feel kind of Rocky Balboa style, doesn't it? But the benefit is real.

How does that sound? Obviously, you don't have to do that all the time. These exercises should be used strategically. The ideal timing would most probably be in the middle of your workout. This is when you have started feeling a little worn out or maybe even bored of the same routine. After warming up and engaging in power stretching, you can bring these moves to the mix and benefit from a toned-up body. So now let's go on to planning your workout routine, shall we? This will help you organize everything and start implementing your working regimen.

Chapter 4: Walking Plan

You have already set realistic goals as to what you want to achieve through walking. You have realized why it is as good an exercise as running, if not better. More than that, you have gone through the essentials you are going to need throughout your workout sessions and you have learned all about how to tone up your upper body, too. And now it is high time you organized stuff and arranged your schedule, including the basics. In this way, everything will be well-thought and you will know exactly what to do.

First of all, where are you going to walk? Are you going to start strolling around the neighborhood or is there a special place you would like to visit? A park nearby, the seaside or an athletic field, they all sound ideal. Be sure to find a place that allows you to relax, take in some fresh air and recharge your batteries, rather than choosing a dull street filled with cars and traffic. This will transform your mood and lift your spirit.

What time are you planning to walk? Are you leaving that to chance? Good luck with that! Unless you set a clear schedule, life is going to get in the way. Before you know it, you will be postponing your walking sessions again and again. Shopping, going out with friends, cooking, taking up way too much time at the office, these are just a few of the excuses you will end up using, so you must have a walking plan, as well as time you can devote to yourself. Maybe mornings work better for you, particularly when during the day you feel drowned by tasks and chores. Wake up a bit earlier, if need be. Alternatively, check the time and frequency that appeals to you the most and stick with that.

Another thing to consider is whether you want to walk alone or you prefer having a walking buddy by your side. There is no right or wrong here. Walking with a buddy motivates you to commit to this activity. You have another person to push you, as well as facilitate the whole process. Talking to somebody can be fun and therefore it is a great option for those who don't want to keep to themselves. Plus, like-minded people always inspire one another and offer constructive advice, suggestions or even a driving force to achieve more.

On the other hand, another person also means that there is a higher risk of distractions. A conversation can drive you off your goals, and you end up enjoying the company of your buddy more and not the benefits of walking. More than that, you need to be sure that your walking buddy coordinates with you and your walking pace. Otherwise, it can be hard to keep up or restrict yourself to wait for them to catch up.

Once every week or so, go through your walking plan and evaluate your progress. Have you managed to stick with the guidelines that you have set? Or maybe you should tweak it up a little to meet your current demands. You have to stay ahead of the game, anticipating that changes will happen. But be ready for them and act accordingly, with tons of flexibility and perseverance.

Changing Walking Speed

Did you know that changing your walking speed can increase the number of calories that you burn by 20% (Stoddard, 2020)? This is amazing! You do not have to dedicate more time in order to shape up sooner. The only requirement is that you act smart and spice it up during your strolls. As a rule of thumb, you should aim at walking at a brisk pace, but alter the speed every five minutes or so, making those muscles burn more and boosting your metabolism. Sprint and then walk slowly before you sprint again. Oh, it should be fun!

Of course, power walking (or speed walking) can work wonders too. Walking at a speed of 7 to 9 kilometers per hour increases the calories you burn and helps you shape up much faster. Although it takes more effort, it tends to be quite addictive (Lindsay, 2018). And bear in mind that you will be walking off the same calories as jogging, if you pay attention. So as soon as you feel confident about your walking performance, try this out and see how it goes. And remember, you can always walk at a slower pace, as long as you remain active.

Variety in speed doesn't only boost performance and promote weight loss. It also prevents you from engaging in a boring workout session that you end up disliking. When something becomes predictable, it can take its toll on the level of determination to commit to such an activity. If there is no suspense as to what happens, if there is no change whatsoever and if there is no element of surprise, well this is not a sustainable option for most people.

By changing your walking speed, you activate different muscles and hence you surprise your body to an extent. As a consequence, your body reacts by burning more calories after having put in motion different muscle groups, so feel free to change your routine as often as possible, trying out various sets of exercises and multiple modifications from brisk walking to a more relaxed pace and vice versa.

What About Walking on a Treadmill?

When you think of the gym, the first image that comes to mind is surely that of people walking or running on treadmills. At the same time, there are many people who choose to invest some money to buy a reliable piece of sports equipment to use at home. A treadmill definitely ranks among the most popular options for working out indoors. But does walking on the treadmill resemble walking outside? And is that workout equally beneficial to you?

First things first. No matter if you select to walk outdoors or on a treadmill, good for you. That being said, there are several factors that make the treadmill less appealing and fruitful for you in terms of weight loss and fitness. When you walk outdoors, you get to walk up and down, with inclines and downhill options that allow you to work different muscles. Treadmills often come with limited options of inclination, but as a general rule they only build specific muscle groups. And the more muscles you work, the more the calories that you burn.

Another disadvantage of treadmills when compared to walking outdoors is the fact that the former costs—the latter doesn't. As simple as that. Moreover, walking outdoors surely lifts your spirit and makes you feel good. You enjoy nature, fresh air, peace and quiet. Instead, walking on the treadmill means that you are facing the four walls of a gym or your home.

Obviously, treadmills do feature some compelling arguments in their favor. First off, you can better control the environment when working out indoors, so you don't have to worry about a heatwave in your town or heavy rain. And it goes without even saying that you can watch TV or even read a book while walking. You cannot do these things outdoors, except for some music using your headphones.

Weigh the pros and cons of each option and decide what's best for you. Treadmills can be affordable, requiring minimal maintenance and keeping you on track. But let's be honest. There is no way treadmills can ever replace the feeling you get when walking outdoors and admiring the magnitude of nature. It is pure magic!

Chapter 5: Shedding Pounds

OK, so you know what to do to keep moving. This is the only way for you to shed some pounds and stay healthy and fit. But is that all? Well, what do you think? Walking can only get you to a certain point when you boost your metabolism, enhance your immune system and start burning more calories for losing weight. Still, you have only scratched the surface. Even though it is vital to incorporate walking in your lifestyle, you have to combine this healthy activity along with a change of dietary patterns. In other words, you ought to change your eating habits and most importantly the ones that would be described as "unhealthy."

Rather than eating junk food and consuming overly processed foods, you should focus on wholesome meals. You can seek advice from a dietician if you think this is all too much for you. But the truth is that you already have the foundations in your head. You simply need to shift your mindset and go for it! "We are what we eat," right? This can be exciting to consider, but it can as well be frightening. Nobody wants to recreate an image in their mind when their very essence is a huge serving of potato chips, deep fried butter and pastries, accompanied by sugary soda drinks. On the downside, so many have associated these food items with their sense of relaxation, entertainment or just chill.

Having committed to a healthier lifestyle through walking is a great step. Now you need to move forward and decide that it is time to take matters into your own hands, 100%! So, picking the right diet plan for you makes sense. This is an essential part of your path to wellness, so you should not decide randomly as to which diet plan is best for you. If you do, you are risking blowing all your hard work away and sabotaging your efforts.

Furthermore, do not listen to the sirens that claim there are magical diets, promising to lose lots of weight in the shortest amount of time. No one has ever lost twenty pounds in a week, following a healthy and sustainable diet. Not only will you jeopardize your health by following an extreme dietary approach, but you will most probably end up gaining the weight back in a jiffy. There are no magic tricks in dieting. So even though there are countless different types of eating plans, you will see that their components are actually pretty much alike.

Implementing the Diet

Every single one of us is different, so it is a no-brainer that you should pick the diet that appeals to you the most.

Otherwise, you will not be able to stick with the plan for long. There are countless options for you to select from, including the Mediterranean diet or a diet that is based on minimal consumption of carbs per day. Whatever ticks the boxes for you is just fine. Just avoid fad diets at all costs! You will most probably suffer and take extreme measures, only to find out that you have gained even more weight after returning to your old patterns.

What you need to opt for is fresh and seasonal fruit and vegetables, lean meat and fish, non-fat dairy and healthy fats of the highest quality standards (Robinson, 2019). This is a generic rule, but it reflects the food options that you should target. On the contrary, you should avoid processed meals, alcohol and sugar, refined wheat and artificial delicacies. Some people prefer to engage in intermittent fasting, as a way to promote weight loss, so if you feel good about it, then you can narrow down your eating window and only consume a couple of meals and a snack, rather than eat five times a day.

Another great tip that you must implement, if you want to maximize weight loss, is the avoidance of drinking your calories. In fact, you will find that most of the time you underestimate the calories found in drinks. A cup of coffee, a refreshing milkshake, a smoothie (no matter how healthy it might appear to be), soda drinks and even fruit juices contain a lot of empty calories. Plus, they do not help you with feeling satiated. As a result, you consume more calories and you still feel hungry and deprived.

As always, planning is the key to success. You must make a plan beforehand and schedule your meals, according to your daily tasks and any events that may come up. For example, if you are having a get-together with colleagues every Friday after work, then you should organize and plan ahead. Make sure that you eat healthy the rest of the day and add a special treat or two during your time with your friends.

A diet should be considered as a way of life and therefore it should be sustainable. You have made some fundamental decisions and you need to find something that meets your criteria, your needs and preferences, let alone your desires. This is the only way you will ever cling to your new diet plan. Make it fun, exciting and adventurous—try out new combos every now and then, do not be afraid of risking and experimenting with different flavors and, no matter what, love yourself for the hard work you are putting in materializing what you have been dreaming of. Congrats!

What About Eating out?

I commend you for being a sociable person, but this doesn't mean that you will throw away all your hard work, simply because you are an extrovert. In other words, you can still enjoy spending time with your family and friends, but you can set your own rules and cling to them. Although at first you might feel like your options are way too limited, over time you will see that this is not true. It is up to you how to look at it. You can focus on what you are deprived of due to your diet plan, or you can choose to look at the silver lining. There is still so much to enjoy, including culinary delicacies and of course, good company and an occasional treat.

As to what you should order when eating out, my advice would be to keep things simple. Every restaurant serves salads, so take advantage of that. Order dressing on the side or ask for olive oil and vinegar instead of creamy sauces. Then, go for grilled meat or fish, along with vegetables (grilled, steamed, boiled, your choice) and avoid unnecessary food like bread and butter, fried appetizers, sugary beverages and so on. Instead, drink your water or request some sugar-free iced tea or a glass of dry wine. As for dessert, why not skip it altogether? If you are craving for something sweet, check out if there is fruit salad. Otherwise, make sure that you split your dessert with someone. What are friends for?

Make smart choices, so as to minimize the effect of a single meal or a night out to your overall effort. Swap the most calorie-dense dishes for lighter versions. Generally, avoid going to places where you used to overindulge. Rather than heading to that Italian place with your favorite pasta, try out Argentinian cuisine for a hearty steak. Or choose Indian over Chinese, if you think that you cannot resist wontons and spring rolls. Furthermore, you can always ask for a kid's menu or half the regular portion of food. Some restaurants have that option, so you can get a taste and not ruin your diet doing so.

There will always be cheat days, when you just don't feel like counting calories or macros and carbohydrates. Plan ahead and make these days special, so that you enjoy good food that fills you up and motivates you to continue with your diet. Remember that you are not a prisoner and this is 100% your own decision. Again, even if you fall, don't forget to get back on your feet. Tomorrow is a new day and you'd better make it a great one!

Chapter 6: The Power of Water in Weight Loss

Do you enjoy some good statistics? Well, the Earth is 71% covered by water and this is a lot! Humans also have a staggering water percentage of their body composition. In fact, a male adult has about 60% water in his body, with the female adult at about 55% and the infant's percentage in water soaring up to the impressive 75% (Helmenstine, 2013). From this, you can pretty much guess why it is essential that you consume enough water to hydrate your body. It helps you stay healthy and it is a true "elixir of life," as many people claim!

As far as weight loss is concerned, water is literally irreplaceable. By drinking water, you boost your metabolism. More specifically, you can burn more calories even when you rest. the only thing that you need to do is drink your water and then enjoy the benefits that come along. And of course, it is needless to say that fat cannot be eliminated without the crucial help of water. How would your body break down fat cells otherwise? More than that, water suppresses your appetite and thus, you had better sip on a glass of water or two whenever you feel hungry. Other pros of water drinking include flushing out toxins and replacing other drinks that can be filled with calories, as mentioned earlier (Johns Hopkins University, 2020).

What about working out? Drinking water is truly helpful to those who engage in any form of exercise. First of all, water allows you to get hydrated and this is very important due to sweating a lot. Water also aids muscles and tissues, as well as your entire body, to function properly and enhances their flexibility and endurance. If you are experiencing leg cramps for example, you should drink more water. And since your lungs and heart work overtime while exercising, water can help a great deal in maintaining their overall health. Buy a fancy refillable water bottle and keep it with you at all times to use before, during and after your workout regimen!

You must have heard about drinking 8 glasses of water per day. How accurate is that? Well, the truth is that this is just an average quantity of water. There are many different factors that determine the exact quantity of water your body needs. Apparently, when you are thirsty you should just have another glass. But, the right amount of water varies according to your weight and your activity level, how much you sweat and even the weather conditions. Thirsty yet?

Tips to up Your Daily Water Intake

Are you having trouble drinking your water every day? Of course, there are many people who love water and don't mind sipping on it throughout the day, reaching their goals and even going the extra mile. However, if you are anything like me, you would rather enjoy other amazing drinks rather than settle for plain water, right? But the truth is that water is life and so you ought to find ways to incorporate it in your daily routine. And by that, I mean figuring out how to drink more water on a daily basis.

Here are some tips that might help you out:

- Use a water bottle and drink water out of it, so that you can keep it close to you and track your progress. Sometimes, when you are in front of the PC screen reading something, you instinctively reach out for the bottle standing right there on the desk. Well, this should become a habit of yours!
- Add flavor to your water. Take some time to slice cucumbers or fruit, tossing them in a water jug. Then add ice and water and stir. Some basil leaves or mint will work wonders, as well as lemon and lime. Sky's the limit, since there are so many combos out there waiting for you to unveil them.
- Download a water tracking app, so as to be reminded of your daily goals. Be realistic, though. You will not make it to the finish line on the first day. Don't give

up! The app will alert you every hour or so, which means that you had better be prepared.

- Instead of drinking plain water, you can opt for sparkling or mineral water. These are both excellent choices. My personal favorite is sparkling water, with some ice and lemon. Find your own treat and enjoy, rather than drink sugary soda.
- An unorthodox method for upping your water intake for the day is to eat salty food. As a result, you will be thirsty and you will want to drink something to quench that thirst. Just keep the water bottle handy, so as not to get carried away and drink up something else.
- Finally, it is a good investment to buy yourself a good water filter. It is important that you drink high quality, clean water, so make sure that you eliminate the threat of dirt and debris, by investing in the water filter. In this way, you can stop worrying about tap water problems.

No matter what you do, push yourself to reach your water goal for the day. Soon, you will become addicted to this watery bliss and you will be surprised as to how quickly you down those bottles that you used to panic over. It is all a matter of habit, so hold on tight!

Do I Need to Drink Just Water?

Although it is recommended that you meet your daily needs in plain water, there are several things that can serve as substitutes. If you enjoy herbal tea, then you will be delighted to hear that you can have as much as you like. Tea is in fact just like water, particularly if you prefer the unsweetened version. More than that, there are countless flavors to pick from, so you are bound to find the one to call your favorite, allowing you to up your daily water intake.

Apart from drinking herbal tea, black coffee can have the same impact. Fruit juices, especially when diluted with some extra water or lots of ice, can work wonders hydrating you. Another drink that can help you out but is considered a mixed blessing is a sports drink. On the one hand, it contains electrolytes and thus allows you to replenish your body. But on the other hand, these sports drinks are only suitable for longer walking sessions that exceed sixty minutes. Be careful not to mistake sports drinks with energy drinks, though.

Even food can help you out with your water consumption for the day. Cucumbers, watermelons, spinach are foods that contain high amounts of water, so if you are trying to increase the water you get from your diet, these are the best options. Plus, you can try out eating more soups and replacing some meals with smoothies or protein shakes.

Typically, water intake features all fluids that you get to consume within the day. Nonetheless, there are better options than sugary soda drinks, per se. So do try to avoid these liquids. They do count towards meeting your daily goals as far as water is concerned, but they do not offer you anything nutrition-wise.

Walking Has Changed My Life

Most people underestimate the power of walking. Everybody walks, so why should it matter so much? In my case, walking has literally changed my life. Back in the day, I always felt tired of getting off that chair and moving around a little. Even the slightest exercise would have me huffing and puffing for hours and that led me to a more introverted lifestyle. Instead of enjoying life with family and friends, I would curl on the sofa and watch TV or read a book. Obviously, there is nothing wrong with that, but when this becomes a habit, then all hell breaks loose.

Extra pounds used to pile up and I suddenly realized that I was overweight and on my way to obesity. It dawned on me that I hadn't even noticed it until I found that my clothes could barely fit. In fact, I used to wear mostly baggy clothes, rather than all the cool outfits that I had bought in the past. My body had not been accustomed to so much weight, which is why I experienced pain all the time. The pain was there, in the back and the joints, in the ankles and the feet. I wasn't always like that and this made me feel so bad. My self-esteem had gone down the drain and instead I felt depressed, isolated and disappointed about my very essence. How could this be? How on Earth did I let it come to this?

Guilt was omnipresent. It was my responsibility to take care of myself and clearly, I had failed so terribly in doing that. I spent so much time regretting things I had done, till one day it hit me. I would change my life, no matter what. Apparently, I needed something drastic. Something that would help me reach my goals, but I did not know where to look. It had to be something simple and easy, so that I could incorporate it into my daily routine without a lot of fuss. Elaborate workouts and extreme diets were not for me. I would start something and soon my enthusiasm would vanish into thin air.

As I was weighing the pros and cons of all sorts of exercise, I realized that none of them would be a viable solution for me. I needed my freedom, without the guidance that a personal trainer or a gym membership would bring. Then, I had to find something that would involve me being outdoors. Rarely do I enjoy being inside a confined space, especially now that I have acknowledged the negative consequences of my past behavior. Another important factor was the cost, as I didn't have many resources at the time and I had to find something really inexpensive. Finally, this exercise would need to be risk-free, since I had put on extra weight and I couldn't handle my body properly.

At first, I was left in absolute agony as to the perfect workout. And out of the blue, I had an epiphany! Walking! This was the one thing I could start right away that didn't require any special equipment or costly subscription. Plus, I would be able to ease my way into walking and gradually increase the speed, along with the effort it takes, and the outcome has been stunning!

Don't think that I dived right in. First, I did some research and tried to comprehend how walking could reverse the situation for me, and then I started experimenting with places to walk, different time frames and durations. I figured out what worked for me best. When I pushed myself to wake up a little earlier in the morning and headed outside for a walk, my day was filled with energy. I was flying and I felt great. On the contrary, sometimes in the evening I would become so lazy that walking seemed like torture. One of the things that helped me whip up the perfect walking training was that I took notes. Even the slightest detail that would appear to be trivial and unimportant. I documented everything and so I was able to make the most out of my walking experience.

I have never felt healthier and happier than I do now. It is a liberating sense that drives you further every step you take. Walking is much more than a workout. It allows you to relax, concentrating on nothing more than your breathing and the beating of your heart. You challenge yourself to push forward and you reach new boundaries, only to outwalk them next time. Though at first, you may barely make it to the finish line, you will soon understand that there is no actual finish line. You keep walking and walking, seeing all those gorgeous results on your body, your mind, your mood and your face...because you are glowing with happiness!

Walking helped me realize how I wanted my life to be. I would try to live a healthy lifestyle and this meant that I would have to say goodbye to some harmful habits. One of them, perhaps my biggest weakness, was treats. Now I had another goal to accomplish. I would stop eating all the foods that made me feel bloated, lethargic and down. Rather than poisoning my body, I would start healing it through a proper diet. And so, I started buying fruits and veggies, rather than pastries and candy. When I could cook a meal at home, I would pick that instead of ordering takeout and putting my body into such an ordeal.

The only way for me to adhere to the diet plan was through walking. This is what drove me to maintain my focus on the goal. I wanted to be healthy and when temptation crept in, I would go out. I would put my shoes on and I would head to my next walking adventure. Every step I took brought me closer to where I wanted to be, where I deserved to be. No fattening meal can ever match that. To be honest, I have slipped once or twice since this journey began. There have been occasions when I enjoyed a chocolate cake or a gelato with friends, whereas in other occasions I sipped on prosecco and had a couple of daiquiris. However, there is nothing holding me back. I don't feel guilt, because I know that I am in this lifestyle forever.

Years have passed since I have set out on this earth-shattering adventure. After having reached my ideal weight and keeping it off for good, after having managed to feel great about myself again, after having seen the tangible results of a healthy lifestyle, I am not going back there. Walking has changed my life, making me see through the fancy wrapping paper of temporary temptations. Walking has changed my philosophy and has allowed me to find the light at the end of the tunnel.

Now I hope that I am able to inspire others through this book to start their own journey. A journey where there will be pain, for sure. There will be doubt and second-guessing. But as the days go by, the destination will get closer and closer. And it is all going to be worth it. Just shift your mindset and get ready to change your life. Start walking and feel the new you shaping up. Take the first step to the rest of your life. You deserve this!

The End

Free Gift

Food For Your Blood Type Chart

https://bit.ly/DroppingWeightWithJustWalkingGuide

Also By Ann Vase

Just Power Walking Essential Guide to Walking for Weight Loss

How Walking Can Help You Lose Weight and Fat

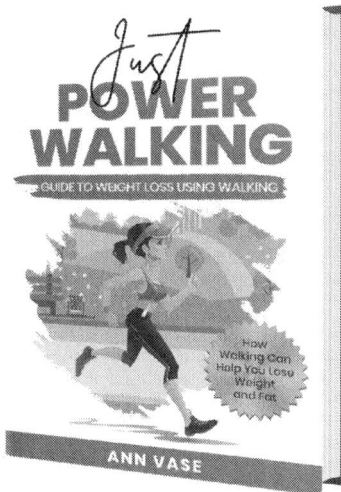

Made in the USA
Monee, IL
28 March 2021